American Ac

DEDICATED TO THE

BLAST!

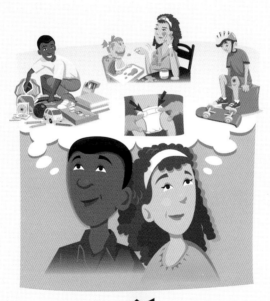

JONES & BARTLETT
LEARNING

World Headquarters
Jones & Bartlett Learning
5 Wall Street
Burlington, MA 01803
978-443-5000
info@jblearning.com
www.jblearning.com

American Academy of Pediatrics
DEDICATED TO THE HEALTH OF ALL CHILDREN®

Robyn R. Wheatley, MPH, Life Support Manager
Wendy Simon, MA, CAE, Director, AAP Life Support Progra
Suzanne N. Brixey, MD, FAAP, Medical Editor
Marilyn J. Bull, MD, FAAP, AAP Board Reviewer

Jones & Bartlett Learning books and products are available through most bookstores and online booksellers. To con
Jones & Bartlett Learning directly, call 800-832-0034, fax 978-443-8000, or visit our website, www.jblearning.com.

Substantial discounts on bulk quantities of Jones & Bartlett Learning publications are available to corporations,
professional associations, and other qualified organizations. For details and specific discount information, contact
the special sales department at Jones & Bartlett Learning via the above contact information or send an email to
specialsales@jblearning.com.

Copyright © 2016 by Jones & Bartlett Learning, LLC, an Ascend Learning Company

The American Academy of Pediatrics and the publisher have made every effort to ensure that contributors to *BLAST!
Babysitter Lessons and Safety Training, Revised Third Edition* materials are knowledgeable authorities in their fields.
Readers are nevertheless advised that the statements and opinions are provided as guidelines and should not be constr
as official American Academy of Pediatrics policy. The recommendations in this publication or the accompanying
resource manual do not indicate an exclusive course of treatment. Variations taking into account the individual
circumstances, nature of medical oversight, and local protocols may be appropriate. The American Academy of Pediat
and the publisher disclaim any liability or responsibility for the consequences of any action taken in reliance on these
statements or opinions.

Production Credits
Chief Executive Officer: Ty Field
President: James Homer
Chief Product Officer: Eduardo Moura
VP, Executive Publisher: Kimberly Brophy
Executive Editor: Christine Emerton
Editor: Alton L. Thygerson, Ed.D., FAWM
Editor: Steven M. Thygerson, Ph.D., MSPH
Associate Acquisitions Editor: Marisa A. Hines
Associate Production Editor: Nora Menzi
Marketing Manager: Jessica Carmichael

Art Development Editor: Joanna Lundeen
Art Development Assistant: Shannon Sheehan
VP of Sales, Public Safety Group: Matthew Maniscalco
Director of Sales, Public Safety Group: Patricia Einstein
VP, Manufacturing and Inventory Control: Therese
    Connell
Composition: diacriTech
Cover Design: Kristin E. Parker
Printing and Binding: John P. Pow Company
Cover Printing: John P. Pow Company

To order this product, use ISBN: 978-1-284-13580-0

The Library of Congress has cataloged the first printing as follows:
BLAST: babysitter lessons and safety training / American Academy of Pediatrics (AAP). — 3e [edition].
    pages cm
  Revised edition of: BLAST : babysitter lessons and safety training, published in 2007.
  Includes index.
  ISBN 978-1-4496-4186-3
1. Babysitting—Juvenile literature. 2. Safety education—Juvenile literature. 3. First aid in illness and injury—Juven
literature. I. American Academy of Pediatrics.
  HQ769.5.B53 2016
  649'.10248—dc23
                              2014024738

6048

Printed in the United States of America
20   10 9 8

Contents

GETTING STARTED

Are You Ready to Care for Children? 5
Sitter Qualities 7
Be Prepared to Answer Questions 7
Be a Good Guest! 8
As They Grow: Ages and Stages 9

SAFETY FIRST

Before Saying "Yes" to a Job 14
A Few Important Points 15
When a Stranger Calls 17
House Rules and Routines 18
Safety Rules 18
Safe House 22
Fire 24
Carbon Monoxide 25
Guns 25

SITTER BASICS

Diapering 26
Bottle Feeding 28
Burping a Baby 30
Feeding a Baby or Toddler 31
Crying 32
Preparing for Bed 34
Behavior Problems 35
Discipline 36
Sitter's Checklist 36

FIRST AID

What to Do for an Injured or Sick Child 39
What Is Not an Emergency? 39
What Is an Emergency? 40
Calling 9-1-1 for Help 40
CPR and Choking Relief 41
Minor Scrapes, Cuts, and
    Open Wounds 48
Bone, Joint, and Muscle Injuries 50
Breathing Difficulty 51
Burns 52
Electrocution 52
Chemical Burns 53
Diabetic Emergencies 53
Diarrhea 54
Dog Bite 54
Eye Injuries 55
Fever 55
Head Injuries 57
Insect Stings 58
Nosebleed 58
Poisoning 59
Seizures or Convulsions 61
Tooth Knocked Out 63
Vomiting 64

FIRST AID KIT

Recommended Supplies 65

KID FUN

Games and Songs 66
Sitter's Busy Bag 70

Getting Started

As a babysitter, parents and guardians trust you with their children's lives. Your main responsibility is to care for a child's needs and keep the child safe. You can prepare yourself for these challenges by following the information in this manual and by completing the BLAST course.

When you are asked by a neighbor, friend, or relative to watch their child, you are being given a job that carries a big responsibility. Sitting is more than a way to earn money.

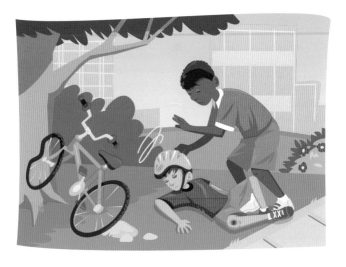

Are You Ready to Care for Children?

- Have your parents or guardians help you decide if you are ready to take on this important job. With their help, you should think about what you will and won't be able

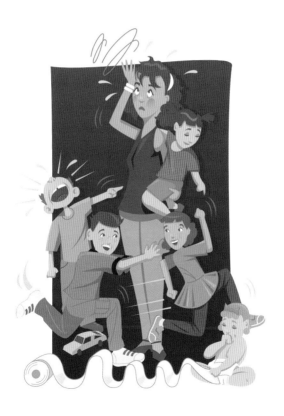

to handle as a babysitter. For example, you may decide to only watch children ages 3 and up or to only work on weekends. Are you mature enough to handle this job? A person must be at least a young adult (12–14 years old) to take on the responsibility of watching young children, and mature enough to handle common emergencies.

- How many children can you handle at one time? A new sitter should start with one child or even start as a mother's helper. A more experienced sitter may handle several children of similar age. It takes a very experienced sitter to handle a mixed age group of children or more than three children at once. Watching too many children can challenge even a very experienced older teen sitter.

- Can you handle babies and young children? Younger teens should not sit for children younger than 6 months. Toddlers can also be challenging. Teens should only accept sitting for one child at a time if the child is three or younger.

- Have you been trained in how to care for small children? Have you received first aid and cardiopulmonary resuscitation (CPR) training from a nationally recognized organization? Discuss with parents or guardians the time frame during which they want you to watch their children, and whether it is proper. Leaving a young child in your care for a few hours is acceptable, but all day or a very late night may not be.

Sitter Qualities

Successful sitters have these
qualities. Are you . . . ?

- Mature
- Trustworthy
- Patient
- Responsible
- Safety-conscious
- Fun-loving
- Punctual

And do you like children?

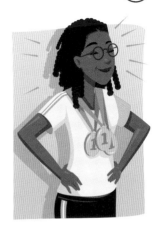

Be Prepared to Answer Questions

Responsible parents or guardians will interview sitters
before hiring them. They want to feel confident that you
can do the job. Expect to be asked the following types of
questions.

Experience

How much babysitting have you done? Have you cared for
other children the same age as theirs? Do you understand the
importance of constantly supervising children?

Training

What training do you have in babysitting and first aid? Do
you know what to do in an emergency?

References

Can you provide names and phone numbers of families who have hired you before? Are you responsible and trustworthy?

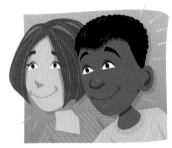

Availability

When can you sit? How late can you sit? What ages of children can you sit for?

Pay

Parents or guardians may ask you what you charge. You should be prepared to tell them a rate per hour that is similar to what other sitters are being paid. You need to determine what sitters are getting paid per hour in your neighborhood. Ask friends who sit and adults who hire sitters what a typical rate is. If the parents or guardians do not ask what you charge, you may politely ask them what they will be paying per hour. It is OK for you to ask how much they will pay you.

Be a Good Guest!

Remember that you are an invited guest in the house. The following rules are good to remember when sitting:

- Only eat food if you have been given permission to do so. If you are welcome to eat, make sure to clean up and wash any dishes when you are done.

- Avoid "exploring" another person's home, such as opening closets or drawers or looking through personal belongings.
- Avoid having friends visit you while you are sitting. This way your attention can always be on the child or children.
- Avoid personal calls or texts. The phone should be kept available for incoming calls from the child's parents or guardians.

As They Grow: Ages and Stages

As children grow older they change. The following table gives information about children as they move through different stages of growth. Remember that this chart is not the same for every child. Some can act differently even if they are the same age and in the same developmental stage.

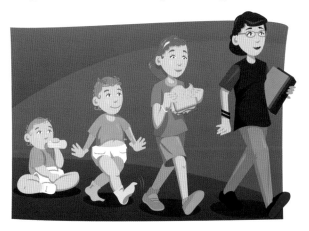

	Infant (0–1 years)	Toddler (1–3 years)
Communication	Responds to sound and touch. Uses eye contact. Begins to mimic sounds. Cries to show tiredness.	Begins to make sounds recognizable as early speech. Responds to tone of voice. Throws tantrums (and objects) when angry. Imitates.
Care	• Change diapers • Bottle or spoon feed • Burp • Hold • Talk to infant	Follow parents' or guardians' guidelines. Help child use the toilet. Spoon feed, but help them feed themselves. Note foods to avoid for this age group on pages 20–21. Help child wash hands and brush teeth.
Safety	Suffocation prevention: Remember the ABC's for sleep: Alone, on their Back, and in a Crib. Always place an infant on its back to sleep in the infant's own crib. NEVER place an infant on a waterbed, beanbag, or anything that is soft enough to cover the face and block air to the nose and mouth. No bedding or soft toys should be placed in the crib.	Investigates everything within reach; very curious. Keep child away from choking hazards. Watch child closely when eating. Limit play space. Never position an infant or toddler in a car seat for feeding, play or sleep. Car seats are only for travel.

(Continues on page 12)

Preschool (3–5 years)	**School Age** (5–8 years)
A 3- to 5-year old has a very large vocabulary. Can say anything he or she wants and often makes five-word sentences. Responds to simple requests.	Can talk with you, but vocabulary probably smaller than yours.
Follow parents' or guardians' guidelines. Let them eat with their hands. Don't force child to eat. Help child use the toilet if needed. Help child wash hands and brush teeth. Will try to comfort you if you are sad.	Should be able to use the toilet alone. Remind them to wash hands afterward and before meals. May want to help you or may have chores to do.
Children are very mobile; limit play area. Monitor their playing.	Know where they are at all times. DO NOT let them do anything that makes you uncomfortable. All children need boundaries.

	Infant (0–1 years)	**Toddler** (1–3 years)
	Never position an infant or toddler in a car seat for feeding, play or sleep. Car seats are only for travel.	
	Burn prevention: Don't heat milk or formula in the microwave. Fall prevention: Don't leave child alone on any furniture, such as a changing table, bed, or sofa (even for a second). Drowning prevention: Don't leave child unsupervised in a bathtub or swimming pool.	
Play	Plays alone with rattles, stuffed animals, and mobiles. Uses eye contact. Reaches and pulls objects. Uses mouth to explore objects.	Curious about never-before-seen items; is possessive of toys (poor sharing). Plays separately from others. May watch others play, but usually won't share or interact. Enjoys being read to and simple games.
Misbehavior	Disciplining not needed. Follow parents' or guardians' guidelines. Does not understand "no."	Use time-out or distraction/restriction. Follow parents' or guardians' guidelines. Does not under-stand "no". Usually responds to "no", but needs redirection and will not remember "no" permanently.

Preschool (3–5 years)	**School Age** (5–8 years)
Enjoys active physical games with interaction (tag, hide and-seek). Enjoys being read to. Imitates adults and playmates.	Enjoys organized games.
Give either/or choices. There may be more success with these than yes-or-no choices. Follow parents' or guardians' guidelines. Understands rules but will test authority.	Can reason with child. Follow parents' or guardians' guidelines.

Safety First

Before Saying "Yes" to a Job

Part of taking a sitting job seriously is protecting yourself as well as the children for whom you will be caring. Know the people you are sitting for before you take the job. Check references if this will be the first time working for this person.

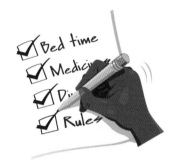

Get the parent's or guardian's name, address, and both home and cell phone numbers. Your parents or guardians may want to meet the people you are sitting for if they are not already acquainted.

Get specific instructions about the number and ages of the children you will be sitting, their bed times, food allergies, medicines, and other information about their personal habits, and what is expected of you. Parents and guardians typically feel confident with a sitter who asks questions and is concerned about the care of their children. Discuss the information with your parents or guardians before accepting the job. Use the Sitter's Checklist (pages 37, 38).

You may find enough jobs simply by letting friends and neighbors know that you are available to babysit. It is not a good idea to post flyers on supermarket bulletin boards or on the street, to place a classified ad in newspapers, or to have a website. You may receive some unwelcomed responses, and it may not be safe. Although most people are nice, do not make it easy for a stranger to find out your age, where you live, or your email address.

Accept jobs only from people you already know or from those who are recommended to you. Accepting jobs from strangers is not as safe as sitting for a neighbor or a neighbor's friend. If you do not know the person calling, ask who recommended you, and tell the caller that you will call him or her back. If you do not know the people you plan to sit for, bring a trusted adult (parent or guardians, adult friend, etc.) along for the interview. The adult is there for support and safety. You should answer any questions and be prepared to ask questions. If you have any doubt or feel uneasy or fearful about the person or situation, refuse the job. Other jobs will become available.

A Few Important Points

- Let your parents or guardians know where and when you are sitting. Always leave the following information with them:
  - Name, address, and phone number of the people for whom you are sitting.
  - Time you will be brought home or need your parent, guardian, or other family member to pick you up from the sitting job.

- Arrange your own transportation to get to the location and to return home. If a family member is not picking you up, call home to let someone know that you are on your way.

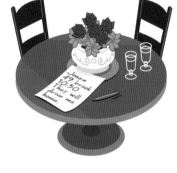

  - Never accept rides from people who have been drinking alcohol or using drugs.
  - Consider creating an agreed-on code word with your family so that if you say, for example, "giggles," they know to come get you right away.
- Be sure you have an escort home. This should be either a parent, guardian, or family member. Never go home alone from a night job.
- Learn how to use the electronic security system if the home has one.
- Let the parents or guardians for whom you are sitting know if you have a curfew. Ask them to call if they are running late.
- Call the child's parents or guardians about a problem such as the following:
  - If a child has been crying for longer than 20 minutes and you can't figure out what's wrong.
  - If a child develops a fever, vomits, or is injured (more than a superficial scrape).
  - Anytime a situation develops that you feel you can't handle without help.

Have a backup plan if you are unable to reach the child's parent. You should also call your own parents or guardians for advice and assistance if something arises.

When a Stranger Calls

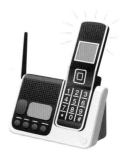

- Always keep the doors locked when caring for a child.
- Never allow strangers into the house unless the parents or guardians specifically informed you that a person would be coming over, such as a neighbor to pick up some items.
- Keep the door closed unless you know the person. Call the police if someone insists on coming in and you do not recognize the person, or if you suspect a prowler. If you must open the door to talk, keep any chain lock fastened until you are sure that it is safe.
- If someone calls, there is no reason to tell a caller that you are a sitter for the children. If you do, this implies that you are alone in the house. If asked, respond by saying that you are visiting, and the parent or guardian cannot come to the phone. Ask to take a message. Tell the caller that the person will return the call shortly.
- Stay inside with the doors locked if you hear suspicious noises or activities outside. Attempting to investigate could be dangerous. Turn on outside lights, and call the police if you suspect a prowler. Be sure that all doors and windows are locked.

House Rules and Routines

Parents or guardians should provide you with each of these items before they leave their children in your care:

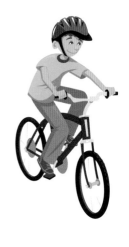

- Acceptable television programs, computer games, and movies
- Food and eating times
- Guidelines for outside play, such as instructions about protective gear (e.g., for bikes, skateboards, scooters, inline skates) and proper clothing, what to do, and where to do it
- Information on allergies or illnesses
- Guidelines for having the children's friends visit
- Bedtime routines
- Special considerations
- Discipline practices—what should you do if a child breaks a rule (time out, to bed early, etc.)
- Rooms off-limits to the children

Note: If the child has an allergy that may require the use of an epinephrine auto injector the parents or guardians should let you know the symptoms the child may show, where the pen is kept and give guidance for its use.

Safety Rules

- Never leave children unattended with small objects. Any food given to children under age 4 should be cut

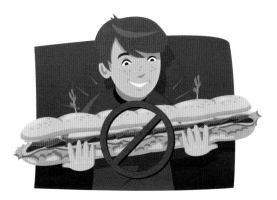

into tiny pieces (about the size of a child's fingertip). Beware of toys that are too small, as the child could choke on the object if swallowed. Any objects left on the floor, such as a coin, can quickly become an object that could choke a child who places it in his or her mouth.

- While holding a baby or young child, you should not eat or drink.
- Medicine should only be given with the parents' or guardians' permission. Follow instructions carefully.
- Be alert when a child is near water. A child should never be left alone in a bathtub. Children can drown in only a few inches of water if they are not watched carefully. A child should never be left alone in a bathtub or pool. Children can drown in only a few inches of water, or even buckets, if they are not watched carefully.
- Have everything you need within arm's reach to bathe a child. (Checklist: soap, shampoo, bath toys, comb, towel, and moisturizer.) If you forgot something or need to answer the phone, take the child out of the water and bring him or her with you.

- Make sure you close all doors and gates to a pool or spa so it is closed off on all four sides to prevent a child from accidentally getting in the water.
- Whenever a child is in or around water there must be someone with strong swimming skills within arm's length providing supervision.
- Always dress children properly for outdoor play activities.
- Keep children away from electrical outlets, stairs, and ovens/stoves.
- Check a sleeping child often.
- Supervise children at all times, especially in the kitchen and bathroom.

Choking Hazards

Food Choking

A little one's airway is about the size of the child's thumb. Any food provided must be cut into tiny pieces to prevent choking. Common food choking hazards include the following:

- Whole grapes
- Raisins
- Popcorn
- Peanuts/nuts
- Hot dogs

- Seeds
- Hard candy
- Raw vegetables

Toy Choking

Babies explore their environment by putting things in their mouths. Never leave small objects that could fit in a child's mouth in their reach, even for a moment. Common toy choking hazards include the following:

- Balloons
- Marbles
- Loose eyes from a stuffed animal
- Small toys, such as game pieces

Objects

- Coins
- Stickers
- Thumbtacks

Safe House

Bedroom 2 – for infant
- Changing table, with one hand used to restrain child. If especially squirmy, put child on the floor on a towel and have all supplies readily available.
- Keep changing table away from windows
- Electrical outlets covered
- Crib, without blankets or pillows.

Kitchen
- Pot handles turned in
- Back burners used
- Hot fluids or food kept out of reach
- Appliances and electrical cords kept out of reach
- Electrical outlets covered
- Cabinets and oven with childproof locks
- Chairs kept away from sink and stove
- Locking trashcan
- Proper highchair for feeding
- Knives and sharp objects put away or protected

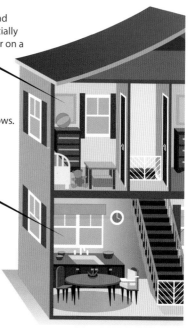

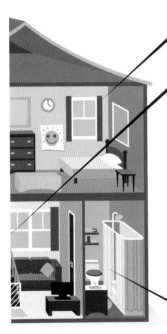

Bedroom 1 – for young child
• Windows or screens secured
• No chairs in front of windows
• Electrical outlets covered
• Small toys or games with small
  pieces stored away

Stairs
• Gates closed and locked at top and
bottom of stairs

Batteries
• Swallowing button batteries is an
  emergency—call 9-1-1 immediately

TV or Furniture Tip Over
• Beware of items or furniture
  toppling off stands

Magnets
• Danger in swallowing
  magnets—medical emergency

Cords
• Keep cords out of reach.
• Beware of accidental hanging or
  strangulation

Bathroom
• Nonskid surfaces
• Locking trashcan
• Cabinets with childproof locks
• Water temperatures set to avoid
  burning
• Appliances and electrical cords
  kept out of reach

Fire

- Plan ahead. Know how to get yourself and the children out of the house in case of fire. Walk through the house with a parent or guardian to ensure all doors and windows are locked and to locate how to leave the house in case of a fire. You should ask the parent or guardian about setting up a prearranged safe meeting place.
- Never let children play with matches, lighters, or fireworks (including sparklers)—these items need to stay out of reach.
- Never leave the stove or oven when cooking.

In Case of Fire or If the Smoke Alarm Goes Off . . .

- Remain calm and think about the exit routes you located previously.
- Sound the alarm—yell "FIRE!" as loud as possible.
- Test doors before you open them. Touch the door with the back of your hand—at the knob and around the frame. If there is a fire on the other side, it will feel warm on the knob and around the cracks. If the door is warm, try another escape route.

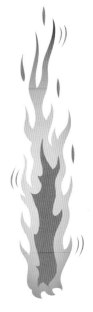

- If possible, close the door to the area where the fire is. Smoke kills, and shutting doors stops it from advancing.
- Leave the fire alone. Attempt to save lives—yours and the children's.
- Get everyone out of the house immediately by staying as low to the ground as possible to avoid smoke inhalation; do not go back in for any reason.
- Keep all the children together. Go to a known neighbor's house or the prearranged safe meeting place.
- Call, or have a neighbor call, the emergency telephone number (usually 9-1-1). Then call the parents or guardians.

Carbon Monoxide

- There should be a carbon monoxide (CO) alarm on every level of the home, especially near sleeping areas.

In Case the Carbon Monoxide Alarm Goes Off . . .

- If the CO alarm sounds, you need to immediately move outdoors for fresh air and then call 9-1-1.

Guns

- A gun can be dangerous if a child tries to play with it. If you come across a gun at the home, follow these safety rules:
  1. Stop.
  2. Don't touch the gun.
  3. Gather the children and leave the area where the gun is.
  4. Tell an adult right away.

Sitter Basics

Diapering

1. Get ready. Have everything you need within reach. Never leave a baby unattended, even for a second. Wash your hands before beginning the procedure.

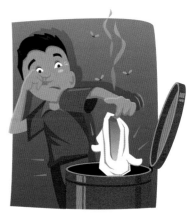

2. Cover the changing surface (crib, floor, or changing table) with a towel or changing cloth. If using a changing table, keep on hand on the child at all times to secure him or her. If the child is especially squirmy, you can place the child on a towel on the floor with all supplies readily available and change them there.

3. Remove the dirty diaper. As you remove the diaper, notice how it was secured. Hold the baby's ankles and carefully lift the hips.

4. Wipe in the correct direction. Using a warm washcloth or baby wipes, gently wipe the baby clean from the front to the back. Wiping from back to front, especially on girls, could spread germs that could cause an infection.

Wipe the creases in the thighs and buttocks. Keep a clean diaper over a baby boy's penis, because he could spray you, the walls, or anything else in range.

5. Dry the baby with a clean washcloth or clean wipe, and apply diaper ointment if needed.

6. Put a clean diaper on the baby by gently lifting the legs and feet and sliding the diaper under the baby. Bring the bottom half of the diaper up through the baby's legs. A boy's penis should be placed downward before fastening the diaper to prevent leaks above the waistline.

7. Fasten the diaper. Bring the adhesive strips of the disposable diaper around and fasten snugly. Avoid sticking the tape onto the baby's skin.

8. Get rid of the diaper. If it is a disposable diaper, empty any bowel movements in the toilet and properly dispose of the diaper. When you get rid of the diaper, be certain not to leave the baby alone on the table!

9. Change any wet or dirty baby clothes.

10. Wash your hands thoroughly after changing a baby's diaper to avoid getting sick.

Be prepared to help toddlers who have recently been "potty trained." They may still need help with undressing, wiping, and washing hands.

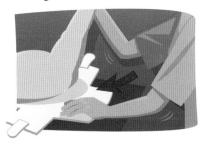

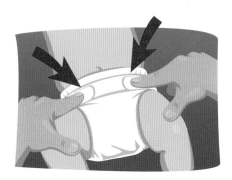

Bottle Feeding

1. Wash your hands before and after feeding the baby. No health reason exists for feeding a baby warmed milk, but most babies prefer it. You can warm a bottle in a pan of hot—not boiling—water or by running it under the hot water tap, or use a commercial bottle warmer if available.

2. A microwave should not be used to heat a milk bottle because the milk does not heat evenly and it can cause burns.

3. Test the milk's temperature by sprinkling a few drops of it on the inside of your wrist before giving it to the baby. If it is too hot on your wrist, it is too hot for the baby.

4. If you offer a bottle and the baby doesn't immediately start sucking, try stroking his or her cheek with your finger. When the mouth opens, insert the nipple completely and make sure it's on top of the tongue, not under it. If the baby isn't awake or alert enough to eat, you can try rousing the baby by sitting him or her up or taking off a layer of clothing to make the baby cooler.

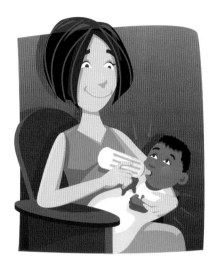

5. The best position for feeding a baby is sitting in an armchair or rocking chair with your elbows and arms supported.

- Make sure the nipple and the neck of the bottle are always filled with breast milk or formula.
- Never force the nipple into the mouth or rattle the nipple in the baby's mouth.
- Switch from one side of the baby's mouth to the other midway through the feed.
- Encourage pauses while the baby drinks from the bottle to prevent the little one from guzzling.
- No need to finish the last bit of milk in the bottle. If the baby releases the bottle nipple before the bottle is empty, he or she is all done.

- If you feel any strain, put pillows under your arms or under the baby until you find a comfortable feeding position. Hold the baby semi-upright in your lap, and cradle his or her head in the crook of your arm. (Make sure the head is higher than the infant's chest. Otherwise fluid can collect in the eustachian tubes and affect the middle ear, causing an ear infection.) Propping the bottle in the baby's mouth can cause tooth decay or choking. Always hold the baby, and keep bottles out of the baby's crib. Hold the bottle so the milk fills the neck of the bottle and covers the nipple. This will prevent the baby from swallowing air as he or she sucks.

Burping a Baby

Even when the flow of liquid is perfect, if babies swallow some air they can become fussy or spit up if they are not burped often. Try burping after the baby takes one-third of the bottle.

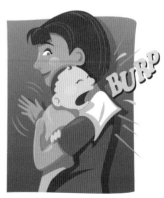

One sign that an air bubble in the stomach may bother the baby is that he or she stops eating before you'd expect him or her to be full. Try these three easy burping methods:

- Hold the baby upright against your shoulder and chest and support the back. Rub, pat, or massage his or her back with your other hand.

- Sit the baby on one side of your lap, support his or her chest with your opposite hand, lean the baby slightly forward, and with your other hand, rub or pat his or her back.
- Lay the baby facedown across your lap—stomach on one leg and the head on the other leg. Support his or her head so it is higher than the chest. Gently rub or pat his or her back.

Feeding a Baby or Toddler

1. Wash your hands before and after feeding the child.
2. Get the food ready before putting the child into the chair or seat. Put the baby food in a dish and put a bib under the child's chin and on his or her chest.
3. Secure the child in the seat with a safety belt if available and lock the tray in place.

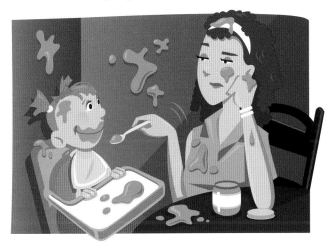

4. Test the food's temperature by sprinkling a few drops of it on the inside of your wrist before giving it to the baby. If it is too hot on your wrist, it is too hot for the baby.
5. Use a small spoon and put about a quarter teaspoonful of food on its tip. If a child doesn't want to eat, that is OK.
6. You may need several spoons in one sitting in case the baby wants to hold on to one or drops one on the ground.
7. Cut all food into thin slices to prevent choking.
8. When finished, wash the child's hands and face, and wipe up any spilled food.

Crying

You can get frustrated when a baby cries, especially if it goes on without stopping. The longer the baby cries, the more difficult the crying will be to stop. Babies cry for many reasons: full diaper, empty bottle, or air in the stomach (keep the baby upright during feeding to reduce air intake). Changing the physical surroundings may help stop the crying. Try one or more of the following methods to get the baby to stop crying:

1. Go for a walk with the baby in a carrier, a sling, or your arms.
2. Rock the baby in your arms, a cradle, a baby swing, or a carriage.
3. Talk to the baby.
4. Cuddle the baby.
5. Sing a song to the baby.
6. Massage the baby's back, arms, or legs.
7. Use a pacifier.
8. Place the baby in the crib or playpen, walk away, and take a few minutes to calm down.

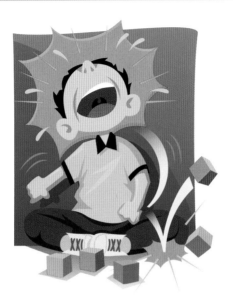

Ask the parents or guardians at what point they would like to be called if attempts to calm the child do not work. You can suggest calling them after 20 to 30 minutes of continuous crying.

Shaken Baby Syndrome

A crying baby can frustrate a caregiver. Do not shake a baby—ever! Babies have very weak neck muscles that are not yet able to support their heads. If you shake a baby, you can damage his or her brain or even cause death. Even a brief period of shaking an infant can damage their brain forever.

Reminder: If you are feeling frustrated with an infant's crying, it is always better to leave the infant in a safe place inside the house and walk away to cool off.

Preparing for Bed

Bedtime can sometimes create anxiety for young children, especially if parents are not home. Here are some tips for making bedtime fun for each age group.

Infants

- Ask the parents or guardians about the usual "bedtime routine" for the baby.
- Gently rub the baby on the back before putting him or her in the crib.
- Lay the baby on his or her back, and take all loose blankets, stuffed toys, or other items out of the crib.
- Play soft music.
- Once the baby is calm, try sitting quietly in the room.
- If the baby cries a lot, help him or her to relax and settle down to sleep.
- Make sure the baby is asleep and turn on the baby monitor and night light before you leave the room.
- Make sure nothing is covering the child's head.

Toddlers

- Ask the parents or guardians the best methods to get the child to sleep.
- Ask parents about bedtime snack before tooth brushing.
- Encourage quiet time as bedtime approaches. Turn off television and radio an hour before bedtime as they stimulate children.
- Make reading or storytelling a fun part of bedtime.
- Stay in the room until the child is asleep.
- Turn on a night light if appropriate.
- Place the door to the room according to the parents' or guardians' and child's request (e.g., leave the door open slightly).

Toddlers and Preschoolers

- Ask the parents or guardians what the child likes to do to get ready for sleep.
- Keep activities calm before naptime or going to bed.
- Read a book together.
- Relax and play imagination games to help the preschooler close his or her eyes.

School-Age Children

- Ask the parents or guardians what time the child should be in bed, and what time he or she should be asleep.
- Older children may want to read or have you read to them before they go to sleep.
- Play soothing music.
- Play imagination games.
- Assure children that their parents or guardians will be home when they wake up in the morning.

Behavior Problems

Children may misbehave for a sitter, even more than for a parent or guardian. Causes for misbehavior include the following:

- Tiredness
- Illness
- Hunger or thirst
- Boredom
- Frustration
- Too much excitement
- Fear
- Need for attention

Discipline

Getting children to behave can sometimes be a challenge.
See the tips in the Sitter's Checklist to help you deal with
discipline issues.

Sitter's Checklist

Give the following checklist to the parents or guardians
ahead of time or let the parents or guardians know that you
will arrive early for them to fill it out.

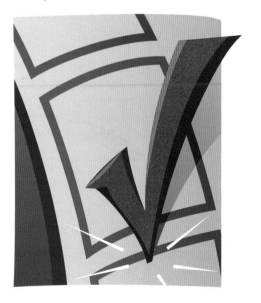

Sitter's Checklist ✔	
Parents' or guardians' first and last names	
House address	
Nearest cross streets or intersection	
House phone number	
Where are the telephones located?	
Where will parents or guardians be?	
When will parents or guardians return?	
Phone number to contact parents or guardians	
You should ask the parents or guardians about a prearranged safe meeting place	
Neighbors' names and phone numbers if parents or guardians cannot be reached	First neighbor: Second neighbor:
Emergency phone number	9-1-1 (if not, it is_____)
Poison Control Center phone	1-800-222-1222
Name and phone number of doctor	
Name and phone number of dentist	
Where are first aid supplies?	
Where is a flashlight?	
How do I lock the door, windows, and security system?	
Where are the best routes out of the house in case of a fire?	
Nightlight on? Yes or No	
Pets' names and care	

Child #1 name Age Nap and/or bedtimes, and usual bedtime routines Special instructions • Food allergies • Medical conditions • Names of medications and dosages • How to help the child in the bathroom • What, how much, and when to feed • Discipline	
Child #2 name Age Nap and/or bedtimes, and usual bedtime routines Special instructions • Food allergies • Medical conditions • Names of medications and dosages • How to help the child in the bathroom • What, how much, and when to feed • Discipline	
Child #3 name Age Nap and/or bedtimes, and usual bedtime routines Special instructions • Food allergies • Medical conditions • Names of medications and dosages • How to help the child in the bathroom • What, how much, and when to feed • Discipline	
Routines to follow	
Rules and restrictions	
Other special instructions	

First Aid

What to Do for an Injured or Sick Child

What Is Not an Emergency?

Some problems need your quick help but are not emergencies. Examples include small cuts, slight fevers, diarrhea or stomachaches, earaches, minor bruises, nosebleeds, rashes, or sprained ankles. You can handle most of these problems yourself. If you are not sure about what to do for a problem that is not an emergency, call the parents or guardians or the child's doctor.

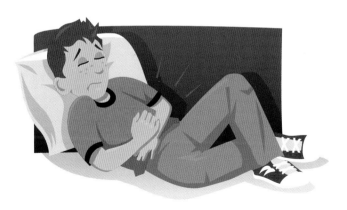

What Is an Emergency?

An emergency is when you believe a severe injury or illness is threatening a child's health or may cause permanent harm. In these cases, a child needs emergency medical treatment right away. Examples of emergencies include the following:

- Unresponsiveness (the child cannot wake up or respond to you)
- Seizures or convulsions (bad shaking that will not stop)
- Choking on food, drink, or an object
- Falls from high places
- Severe burns
- Trouble breathing
- Eating or drinking something poisonous
- Heavy bleeding that will not stop
- Cannot move arms or legs

Calling 9-1-1 for Help

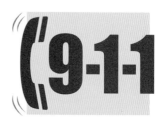

Any time you think a child is in danger, immediately call the emergency telephone number (9-1-1 in most cities and towns) for help. Be ready to tell the 9-1-1 dispatcher the following information:

- Your name and the phone number you are calling from
- What happened and who it happened to
- Exact address of the emergency and the closest major cross streets or intersection

Wait for the dispatcher to hang up. The dispatcher may keep you on the line and be able to tell you how to care for the child until the ambulance arrives.

After you have called your local emergency medical service (EMS), contact the child's parents or legal guardians.

CPR and Choking Relief

CPR and Choking

For a child or infant not moving, use the letters **RAP-CAB** to remember what to do. Start as soon as possible!

R = Responsive? Tap the child or infant and shout, "Are you OK?"	
If child or infant …	**Then…**
Does not move, moan, or answer and is not breathing or is only gasping (sounds like a snort, snore, or groan)	CPR is needed. Go to step **A = Activate.**
Moves, moans, or answers and is breathing	Place on his/her side and keep checking the child or infant. Go to step **A = Activate to call 911 – no CPR needed.**
A = Activate the emergency medical service (EMS) by calling 9-1-1.	
If…	**Then…**
You are alone with an unresponsive child/infant	Initiate CPR then after 5 sets (or 2 minutes) of 30 compressions and 2 breaths, call 9-1-1.
Another person is available with you and an unresponsive child/infant	Send him/her to call 9-1-1 and get AED if available while you start CPR with 2 minutes of 30 compressions and 2 breaths.
P = Position on his/her back and on a firm, flat surface	
C = Chest compressions. Push hard and fast	

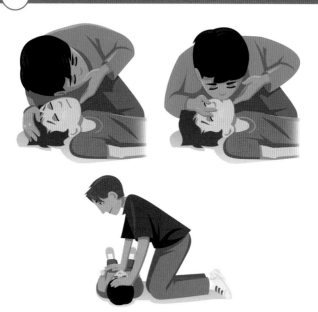

Where to place hands?	How deep? Push hard!	How fast? Push fast!	How many?
For child: Use 1 or both hands—If using 1 hand place the heel of hand on the breastbone in center of chest. If using 2 hands, place one hand on the chest with the other hand on top and interlock fingers to keep them off the chest.	**For child:** about 2 inches; **For infant:** about 1½ inches. Push straight down. Allow chest to come back up to its normal position after each compression.	Push chest at same beat of the Bee Gee's song "Stayin' Alive." Count at fast rate: "1, 2, 3, 4, 5…30." At least 100-120 per minute.	Give 30 compressions without interruption.

For infant: use 2 fingers with one touching and both below imaginary line nipple.

A = Airway open. Open airway by tilting head by pushing forehead back and lifting chin.

B = Breaths. Give 2 normal breaths (1 second each) that make chest rise.
For child: Pinch child's nose shut, cover the child's mouth with your mouth, making an airtight seal. Use CPR mask if available.
For infant: Cover infant's mouth and nose with your mouth, making an airtight seal. If this does not work, try either the mouth-to-mouth or mouth-to-nose technique.

If...	Then...
2 breaths make chest rise	Continue CPR: • 30 chest compressions (push hard and fast). • 2 breaths (1 second each). Take a regular breath, not a deep breath, between the 2 breaths. • DO NOT stop to check for breathing until after every 5 sets of compressions and breaths.
First breath does not make chest rise; the airway may be blocked.	Retilt head, give a second breath: • If second breath does not make chest rise, continue CPR. Each time the airway is opened to give a breath, look for an object in the mouth and, if seen, remove it.

Continue CPR until:
• Victim begins breathing, speaks, or moves
• You are replaced by a trained person
• You are physically exhausted and unable to continue

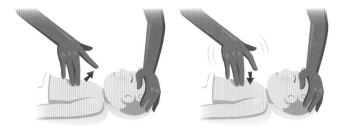

Hands-Only CPR

If you have no CPR training, are unsure about what to do, or unable to give breaths for any reason, at least do the following:

1. Call 9-1-1 or other local emergency number for help.
2. Give chest compressions only. Push hard and fast in the center of the chest. Refer to the above chart about how to give chest compressions.

Choking Child

What to Look For	What to Do
• Coughing loudly and makes some sounds. • Nods head "yes" when asked if he/she is choking.	Let the child cough while you watch for signs of no improvement.

- Is responsive but not coughing or making any sound.
- Is not breathing
- Grabbing or clutching at throat (the choking sign)

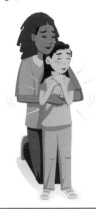

1 Stand or kneel behind the child and wrap your arms around the child's waist with your hands in front.
2 Make a fist with 1 hand and place the thumb side slightly above child's belly button (navel) with your knuckles up.
3 Grab the fist with your other hand and press fist into the child's abdomen with quick, upward thrusts
4 Continue giving thrusts until:
- The object comes out,
- The child starts coughing, talking, and/or breathing,
- You are replaced by a trained person, or
- The child becomes unresponsive (in this case, go to the next step below).

Becomes unresponsive

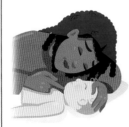

1 Place the child on a firm, flat surface and give 30 chest compressions.
2 Open the airway and look for an object. Try to take it out only if you see an object in the mouth.
3 Give 2 breaths. If first breath does not make chest rise, retilt head, and give a second breath. If second breath does not make chest rise, give 30 compressions

followed by 2 breaths. Before each set of 2 breaths, check the mouth for objects. Only if you see an object in the mouth should you try to take it out.

4 Call 9-1-1 after 5 sets of 30 compressions and 2 breaths.

5 Continue giving sets of 30 compressions and 2 breaths until:
- The object comes out,
- The child starts coughing, talking, and/or breathing,
- You are replaced by a trained person.

Choking Infant

What to Look For	What to Do
Coughing loudly and making some sounds	Let the infant cough while you watch for signs of no improvement.

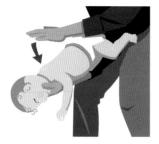
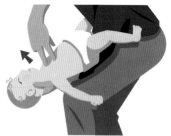

Is responsive but is not crying, breathing, or coughing	1 Hold infant's head and neck with one hand by supporting infant's jaw between your thumb and fingers. 2 Place infant face down over your forearm with head lower than his/her chest. Brace your forearm and infant against your leg. 3 Give 5 back blows between the infant's shoulder blades with the heel of your free hand. 4 Turn infant face up while supporting head. 5 Give 5 chest compressions using 2 fingers over the breastbone as you would in giving CPR but at a slower rate. 6 Repeat 5 back slaps and 5 chest thrusts until: • The infant breathes, coughs, or cries, • You are replaced by a trained person, or • The infant becomes unresponsive (in this case, go to the next step below)
Becomes unresponsive	1 Place the infant on a firm, flat surface (such as a table) and give 30 chest compressions. 2 Open the airway and look for an object. Try to take it out only if you see an object in the mouth.

for objects. Only if you see an
object in the mouth should you try
to take it out.

4 Call 9-1-1 after 5 sets of 30 compressions and 2 breaths.

5 Continue giving sets of 30 compressions and 2 breaths until:

- The object comes out,
- The infant starts coughing, talking,
and/or breathing,
- You are replaced by a trained
person.

Minor Scrapes, Cuts, and Open Wounds

1. Look carefully to see where the blood is coming from.
   Wear medical gloves if you can or protect your hand with
   a wad of paper towel or other clean material.
2. Press steadily on the wound for 5 minutes with a sterile
   dressing or clean, dry cloth.
   - If bleeding is from an arm or leg, raise the arm or leg while
     still pressing on the wound, unless the arm or leg is broken.
3. If bleeding is easy to control, rinse the wound with clean
   running water.
   - Apply a Band-Aid. Remember that small plastic-backed
     Band-Aids are a serious choking hazard for children
     younger than 3 years, so use dressings made of fabric
     instead.

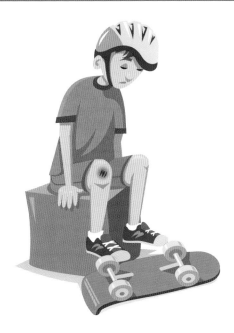

4. If bleeding is hard to control or the wound is still bleeding after 5 minutes, then call the parents or guardians or 9-1-1.
   • While waiting for help, have the child lie on his or her back, raise the child's legs 8 to 12 inches, and keep the child warm with blankets.
5. Shallow wounds can be washed with clean, running water.
   • Apply a bandage and follow up with the parents or legal guardians.

6. For a deep wound, do not try to clean the wound or apply antibiotic ointment.
   - A deep wound requires cleaning by a medically trained person. Call the parents or guardians and 9-1-1.

Bone, Joint, and Muscle Injuries

The injury is probably minor if:

1. it does not interfere with movement OR
2. it is limited to fingers and toes that are not deformed.

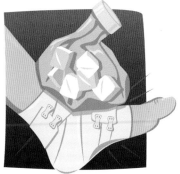

   - Use RICE for care:

   R = Rest: Keep the body part in place and out of use.

   I = Ice: Cover the injury with a wet cloth and apply ice or a cold pack for periods of 20 minutes every 2 hours.

   C = Compression: When not applying an ice bag, wrap an elastic bandage around the body part if one is available.

   E = Elevation: Raise the injured body part above the heart level by placing the injured limb on several pillows.

   - Call the parents or guardians or a neighbor.

The injury is probably more serious if:

1. a deformity is present OR
2. the child won't move the body part and it involves more than fingers or toes.

If you suspect a broken bone or injured joint:

- Keep the body part in place.
- Stabilize the part by holding it still.
- Call 9-1-1 and the parents or guardians or a neighbor.

Breathing Difficulty

For Asthma

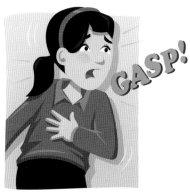

Any child who has asthma and says he or she feels short of breath or begins coughing or wheezing will need your intervention. If a child has asthma, make sure the family shares with you the child's asthma action plan and specifies what medicine the child needs and how to administer it before leaving the child in your care.

1. Keep the child upright.
2. Have the child take slow, deep breaths through the mouth while administering the medication to the child.
3. If the child has a doctor-prescribed handheld inhaler, give it to the child. He or she will know how to use it.
4. Call the parents or guardians.

Burns

1. Apply cool water or cool, wet cloths.

If...	Then...
minor burns (red skin), such as from a sunburn	• apply a clean, dry gauze pad over the burned area. • do not apply burn ointments or petroleum jelly to the burn. • do not break any blisters.
severe burns (blisters, discolored skin)	• call 9-1-1 and parents or guardians or neighbor.

Electrocution

If...	Then...
child is still touching wire, appliances, etc.	turn off the power source before you touch the child so you do not become electrocuted.
the child is unresponsive	use the methods described in the CPR section. Call 9-1-1.
the child is responsive	call parents or guardians.

Chemical Burns

1. Wear medical gloves to protect yourself from contact with the chemical.
2. Flush with running water for about 15 minutes (until an ambulance arrives).
3. Call 9-1-1 and parents or guardians or neighbor.

Diabetic Emergencies

The parents or guardians should tell you if their child is diabetic. Before leaving, the parents or guardians should also tell you how to recognize and handle a diabetic emergency. Suspect an emergency if the child starts to mumble, fumble, stumble and is not alert.

1. If the child is old enough, ask the child to check his or her blood sugar, and then call the parents with the results.
2. If the child cannot check blood sugar, but can swallow, give some food or drink containing sugar. Examples: table sugar, soda, or fruit juice.
3. If not better in 10 to 15 minutes, give the child more sugar and call parents or guardians. If unresponsive, call 9-1-1.

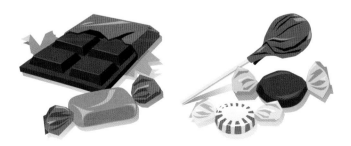

Diarrhea

Diarrhea is frequent, watery, mushy stool and can have several causes. Have the child drink lots of fluids.

1. Most children should continue eating a normal diet, including formula or milk, while they have mild diarrhea.
2. Some children are not able to tolerate cow's milk when they have diarrhea, and it may be temporarily removed from the diet.
3. If the child wears diapers, change them immediately and clean the child after each diarrhea episode. Apply petroleum jelly. Wash your hands after every diaper change or toilet assistance.

Dog Bite

Take caution around family pets. Follow these rules to keep yourself and the children safe:

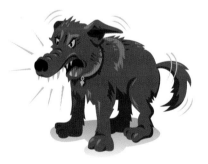

- Children should not be left alone in a room with a dog.
- Keep children away from eating or sleeping dogs.
- Children should not tease or hurt dogs.
- Toddlers should not play close to a dog. Toddlers fall easily and might fall on top of the dog. Even gentle dogs snap when they have been startled or hurt.
- If a dog scares you, you can refuse to sit for the family.

In Case of Dog Bite

1. Place a sterile dressing or clean, dry cloth over the bite site.
2. Press on the wound to stop bleeding.
3. Wash the bite wound with soap and water for 5 minutes.
4. Cover the bite wound with a sterile dressing or clean cloth.
5. Call the parents or guardians or a neighbor.
6. If the animal is unknown, get a good description of it.
7. If the animal is a family pet, put it in a room by itself.

Eye Injuries

If...	Then...
a loose object (eyelash, dust, dirt, etc.) is in the child's eye	gently grasp the upper lid and pull it out and down over the lower eyelid. Tears that occur when you pull the upper lid over the lower lid may help dislodge the object.
an object is stuck in the child's eye	call 9-1-1. Leave the object where it is. Call the parents or guardians or neighbor. Attempt to cover the injured eye with an eye shield or paper cup.
chemical is in child's eye	flush the eye with lukewarm water for 15 to 20 minutes. Call the parents or guardians or neighbor.

Fever

Fever—a high body temperature (over 98.6°F)—is developed by the body to fight an infection. A fever in a child younger than 3 months needs medical attention. Fever can cause a seizure that can be frightening but does not usually result in serious problems.

If the child is younger than 3 years, taking his or her temperature with an axillary (armpit) thermometer is recommended. Taking an oral temperature is not recommended for young children because they cannot hold the thermometer under the tongue with the mouth closed. Ear thermometers are acceptable, though not for children younger than 4 months.

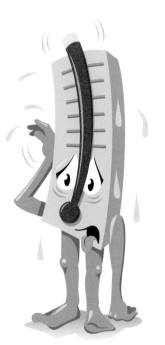

To help reduce fever:

1. Dress the child in light clothing, but do not allow the child to shiver. Shivering increases the body temperature.
2. Bathing with lukewarm water helps bring down fever. Cold water or rubbing alcohol should not be used to bathe a child.
3. If the temperature is above 101°F, call the child's parents or guardians.
4. Aspirin should not be given to a child.
5. Do not provide acetaminophen or ibuprofen unless you have spoken with the parents or guardians.

Head Injuries

If...	Then...
bleeding from scalp	apply gentle pressure to control any bleeding. Call parents or guardians or neighbor. For a shallow scalp wound, flush with water from a faucet. Wear medical gloves if you can or protect your hand with a wad of paper towel or other clean material. Press steadily on the wound for 5 minutes with a sterile dressing or clean, dry cloth. Put a clean bandage on the wound once the bleeding has stopped. After dressing, apply ice pack for 15 to 20 minutes to help with pain and swelling.
swelling appears and is painful	apply ice pack for 15 to 20 minutes (even if swelling is not obvious).
child does not move	see CPR section. If breathing, place child on left side to keep airway open, to drain fluids, and to handle possible vomiting.

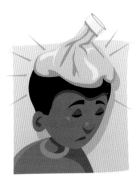

Insect Stings

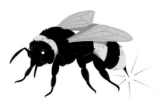

If the child has a known allergy to insect stings and has a doctor-prescribed epinephrine auto injector, a parent or guardian should let you know where the pen is kept and give guidance for its use before leaving the child in your care.

1. Wash stung area with soap and water.
2. Remove any stinger or part of the biting insect by scraping it with a credit card or finger nail.
3. Wash stung area with soap and rinse well with water.
4. Cover the area with a cloth and apply ice for 15 to 20 minutes. Do not put ice directly on the skin.
5. Call 9-1-1 if the child is having difficulty breathing or swallowing.
6. If the child is known to be allergic to insect stings and has a doctor-prescribed epinephrine auto injector use it. Then call 9-1-1 and the parents.

Nosebleed

1. Keep child in sitting position leaning slightly forward. Remind child to breathe through the mouth.
2. Wear medical gloves if possible and use the thumb and finger of one hand to pinch the lower soft parts of the nose together.
3. If bleeding continues for more than 30 minutes, call parents or guardians or neighbor.

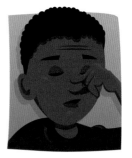

Poisoning call 911 first

Poisoning is one of the most common childhood injuries. Children between the ages of 8 months and 6 years are the most likely to be poisoned. Poisons can look like things that are good to eat and drink. They can come in many colors and forms, including solids, liquids, sprays, or gases. Young children are curious. They like to put things in their mouths, especially if they look colorful or smell nice.

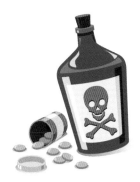

Some common poisons found in and around the home:

- Medicines
- Cleaning products
- Batteries
- Cigarettes
- Plants (indoor and outdoor)
- Iron pills
- Laundry products
- Bug and weed killers
- Alcohol
- Mouthwash

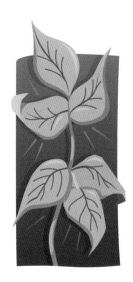

Avoid problems by:

- Keeping children where you can see them at all times, even when you go to answer the telephone. Never leave young children alone, even for just a minute!
- Placing all medicines and household cleaning products out of the reach and sight of children. Keep poisons off of counters.

In case of poisoning:

1. Take action immediately. Have the Poison Control number (1-800-222-1222) by the phone or preprogrammed into your cell phone. Some of the questions you may be asked include the following:
   - What and how much poison the child swallowed (have the container with you)
   - What kind of plant the child swallowed or touched (have a sample with you, such as leaves, flowers, or berries)
   - When the poisoning happened
   - Child's age and weight
   - Child's allergies and medical conditions
   - Child's signs and symptoms
2. If the child has trouble breathing, has seizures, or won't wake up, call 9-1-1 or the local emergency telephone number. Call the parents or guardians in all cases.

If...	Then...
responsive	call Poison Control.
unresponsive	call 9-1-1 and then begin CPR if needed.
a poison is splashed on the skin or in **the eye(s)**	rinse skin/eye(s) with warm running water for 20 minutes. Take off any splashed clothing. Call the Poison Control Center at 1-800-222-1222.
a poison is **breathed in**	get into fresh air; open doors or windows. Call the Poison Control Center at 1-800-222-1222.
cleaning product or substance causes burning sensation or is swallowed	call the Poison Control Center at 1-800-222-1222. Under the Poison Control Center's advice, you may give the child one glass of water or milk to drink (unless the child is unresponsive, has convulsions, or is unable to swallow). Call 9-1-1.
a child swallows a battery or magnet	Call 9-1-1.
anything else is swallowed	call the Poison Control Center at 1-800-222-1222. Keep the child on his or her left side to delay the movement of the poison into the small intestine where it can damage the body faster. Keep the child from eating or drinking before calling the Poison Control Center.

Seizures or Convulsions

If a child is prone to seizures, ask the parents or guardians for guidance about what to do and who to call before they leave the child in your care.

Causes of seizures, other than a seizure disorder (epilepsy), include high fever, head injury, serious illness, and poisoning.

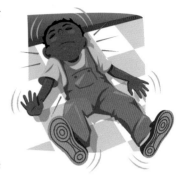

1. Allow the seizure to occur and do not restrain the child's movements.
   - Clear the area to make sure the child won't be hurt.
   - Cushion the child's head with something soft, such as a towel.
2. If possible, roll the child onto his or her left side.
3. Nothing should be forced between the child's teeth. The child should not eat or drink until fully alert.
4. After the seizure stops, keep the child on his or her side to rest. Recovery is slow and the child will sleep or be drowsy for a while.
5. Always notify the parents or legal guardians when a seizure occurs.
6. Most seizures are NOT emergencies and will not require medical help. IF any of the following conditions occur, you should call 9-1-1:
   - The child turns blue or is not breathing.
   - The seizure lasts more than 5 minutes or a second seizure starts.
   - You have not been told that the child is subject to seizures.
   - Any signs of injury or sickness are seen.

Tooth Knocked Out

A child's teeth begin to appear at about 6 months of age. By age $2^{1/2}$ all teeth will have appeared. These are "baby" teeth. Permanent teeth replace the first set of teeth beginning at about age 6 and continue until about age 17.

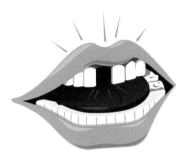

If...	Then...
a tooth has been knocked out	position the child so that bleeding does not cause choking. Stop the bleeding with sterile gauze and direct pressure. Pick up the tooth by the crown (the chewing part), not the root. Gently rinse the tooth with water. Be gentle. Avoid the following: a. Soap or chemicals b. Scrubbing the tooth c. Drying the tooth Gently place the permanent tooth back in its socket. If the child is able to assist, ask him or her to hold the tooth in place with a finger or tissue. Do not attempt to reinsert a primary or baby tooth. If the child is too young to hold the tooth in place or is upset, or if reinserting the tooth is not possible, place the tooth in egg white or coconut water, or if those are unavailable, milk, saline solution (1 teaspoon of table salt added to 8 ounces of water), or water. The tooth should be carried with the child to the dentist. Call parents or guardians immediately. It is best for the child to be seen by a dentist within the first 30 minutes after the tooth has been knocked out.

Vomiting

Vomiting is common in children and may be caused by several things. It usually is not serious and quickly passes. Occasional vomiting is not a cause for worry.

1. Children should not eat or drink for 1 hour after vomiting.
2. After 1 hour of stomach rest, provide small, increasing amounts (0.5 to 2 oz) of fluid every 20 minutes for four feedings. If the child begins vomiting again, allow the stomach to rest for another 30 minutes and then start over.
3. Call the parents or guardians if any of the following conditions are true:
   - The child is an infant younger than 6 months.
   - The child is unable to keep any fluid in the stomach for several hours.
   - The child shows signs of dehydration, such as dry lips and mouth, a dry diaper for several hours, or small amounts of deep gold-colored urine.
   - The child has severe abdominal pain.
   - There is blood or dark green in the vomit.
   - The child looks or acts very ill.

First Aid Kit

Recommended Supplies

The parents or guardians may have a first aid kit in their house. However, you should take a small first aid kit along with your other sitter supplies. You can make your own or buy one. Keep children away from the kit. Some of the contents can be dangerous. Suggested first aid supplies:

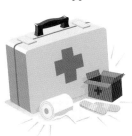

- Elastic wrap (2-inch) for wrapping joint and muscle injuries
- Scissors with rounded tips
- Adhesive tape to hold dressings in place
- An instant cold compress
- Dressings (2-inch sterile gauze pads) and adhesive strips of various sizes for covering cuts and scrapes (children like the ones with designs)
- Hydrocortisone ointment (1%) for rashes that itch
- Tweezers to remove small splinters
- Thermometer (digital; nonmercury and nonglass) for measuring fever in children 5 years and older
- Medical exam gloves (disposable) to protect your hands from blood and reduce chance of infection (two pairs)
- Face shield or face mask
- Small flashlight
- This manual
- Completed Sitter's Checklist (pages 37, 38) or a list of emergency phone numbers

Games and Songs

Using these ideas depends on the child's age.

- Draw or color. Bring scrap paper for drawing, and coloring books. Use crayons or washable markers.
- Play a child's audiotape or CD of something fun and lively. Start dancing around the room.

Children love to play games. Using these ideas depends on the child's age.

- 20 Questions
- Ring Around the Rosy (words are found in the song section)
- Hide-and-Seek
- Simon Says
- Mother May I?
- I Spy

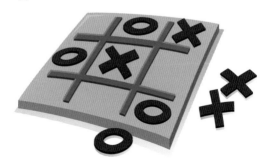

- Play zoo. Have one person pick an animal and act like it while the others guess what animal the person picked.
- Go outside and look at the clouds. Describe them to each other and try to get the others to see which one you're looking at.
- Buy inexpensive books of (1) dot-to-dot, (2) mazes, (3) crossword puzzles, (4) stickers.
- Hangman
- Tic-Tac-Toe
- Tag
- Get children lined up by a mirror and make faces; see who can make the scariest, silliest, ugliest, and happiest faces.
- Children love when you read to them. Read nursery rhymes from well-known books, such as those of Dr. Seuss or Winnie-the-Pooh. Your local library may have these and many more.
- Children love music. They enjoy singing fun little songs. Here are some words to some all-time favorites.

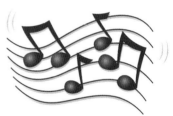

Bingo

There was a farmer had a dog
And Bingo was his name
B-I-N-G-O . . . B-I-N-G-O . . . B-I-N-G-O
And Bingo was his name
   (Spell out B-I-N-G-O)

Head and Shoulders, Knees and Toes

Head and shoulders, knees and toes, knees and toes,
Head and shoulders, knees and toes,
Eyes, ears, mouth, and nose,
Head and shoulders, knees and toes, knees and toes.
(Point to each part of body, repeat song, stop singing a
    part of the body on each repetition but still point to it.
    Keep going until not singing anymore, only pointing.)

If You're Happy and You Know It

If you're happy and you know it clap your hands.
    [clap, clap]
If you're happy and you know it clap your hands.
    [clap, clap]
If you're happy and you know it and you really want to
    show it,
If you're happy and you know it clap your hands.
    [clap, clap]
If you're happy and you know it stomp your feet…
    [stomp, stomp]

Row, Row, Row Your Boat

Row, row, row your boat
Gently down the stream
Merrily, merrily, merrily, merrily
Life is but a dream.
(This song can be sung as a "round." Group 1 starts
    the song;
Group 2 starts when group 1 is finished singing the
    first line.
Group 2 will be the last group singing by themselves.)

Ring Around the Rosy

(Children join hands, go around in a circle)
Ring around the rosy
Pocket full of posies
Ashes, ashes
We all fall down!
(Everyone falls down)

Twinkle, Twinkle, Little Star

Twinkle, twinkle, little star,
How I wonder what you are.
Up above the world so high,
Like a diamond in the sky.
Twinkle, twinkle, little star,
How I wonder what you are!

Old MacDonald Had a Farm

Old MacDonald had a farm, E-I-E-I-O.
And on this farm he had a cow, E-I-E-I-O.
With a "Moo, Moo" here and a "Moo, Moo" there,
Here a "Moo," there a "Moo," everywhere a "Moo, Moo."
Old MacDonald had a farm, E-I-E-I-O.
Old MacDonald had a farm, E-I-E-I-O
And on his farm he had a _____.

Patty Cake

Patty cake, patty cake, baker's man
Bake me a cake as fast as you can.
Roll it and pat it and mark it with a "B"
And put it in the oven for baby and me.

Itsy Bitsy Spider

Itsy bitsy spider went up the water spout.
Down came the rain and washed the spider out.
Out came the sun and it dried up all the rain.
And the itsy bitsy spider went up the spout again.

Sitter's Busy Bag

This can include items that are fun activities for children.
Choose things appropriate for the age of the child or children

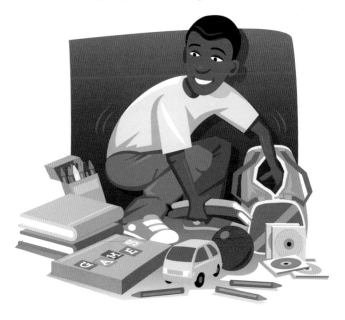

you are sitting. Avoid choking hazards—anything little ones can put fully in their mouths. Place the items in a container (such as a shoe box or a sports bag) to carry them. Suggested Busy Bag items include the following:

- Rubber animals
- Plastic or wooden animals with smooth edges
- Soft plastic- or cloth-covered books
- Plastic or wooden toy cars or trucks with no small detachable parts
- Large rubber ball
- Books: nursery rhymes, stories, coloring, dot-to-dot, mazes
- Crayons, washable markers
- Paper (scrap)
- Words to children's songs (see songs in this manual)
- Games
- Music

Quick Index

Asthma   51

Bedtime   34

Bleeding   48

Blisters   52

Bone injuries   50

Breathing difficulties   51

Burns   52

Burping baby   30

Checklist (Sitter's)   36

Convulsions   61

Crying   32

Diabetic emergencies   53

Diapering   26

Diarrhea   54

Discipline   36

Dog bites   54

Electrocution   52

Eye injuries   55

Feedings

   Bottle   28

   Spoon   31

Fever   55

Fire emergency   24

First aid kit   65

Games   66

Guns   25

Head injuries   57

House rules   18

Insect stings   58

Joint injuries   50

Muscle injuries   50

Nosebleed   58

Poisoning   59

Safety rules   18

Seizures   61

Sitter's Checklist   36

Songs   66

Strangers   17

Swallowed poison   59

Tooth injuries   63

Vomiting   64